# Acupuncture

*Users Guide for Healing Diseases naturally*
*Natural Medicine for Treating &*
*Healing Diseases*

GRACE J. ALLEN

# T a b l e   o f   C o n t e n t s

# Table of Contents

# Introduction

*Did you ever wonder how acupuncture works?* This book strips away the mystery. Each acupuncture point has unique functions, which are explained in plain English for the non-acupuncturist.

Acupuncture functions by stimulating the discharge of endorphins, your body's natural pain-relieving chemicals, it also affects the autonomic nervous system and the release of chemicals that regulate blood circulation and pressure, reduces swelling, and calm the mind.

Acupuncture is a regular Traditional Chinese medication (TCM) practice that originated a long time ago. It is predicated on the premise of a blockage or disruption in the circulation of your body's *life energy or "Qi"*; this can cause medical issues.

Relating to TCM theory, there are over 1000 acupuncture factors on your body, each laying on a low profile energy route, or "meridian"; each meridian is associated with a different body organ system.

*How to do acupressure effectively to treat yourself. This book explains which points are the best to treat different ailments. Acupuncture treats pain, stress, fatigue, emotional disorders, insomnia, digestive problems, and many internal disorders.*

# Chapter 1

## What's Acupuncture?

Acupuncture is a recovery technique that originated a lot of years back from traditional Oriental medication (TCM). This practice would depend on the theory an imbalance in energy triggers medical ailments and mental health disorders. TCM theories proves that the body contains essential life energy called chi; whenever your body and brain will work correctly, chi should undertake the body's vigour stations. These stations are called meridians and may be bought at sure factors during your body. Based on the custom, sometimes chi becomes congested in a variety of meridian pathways, leading to disease or disorders.

The goal of acupuncture is to regenerate the medical and balance from the channels. During acupuncture treatment classes, small needles sit along with specific areas of the body. Known as acupuncture factors, these areas are often where blockage of energy could be happening. The needles can be found in many thicknesses and sizes.

Until the overdue 1990s, acupuncture needles weren't named tools to deal with medical ailments. In 1997, the U. S. Food and Medication Administration (FDA) approved the use of acupuncture needles as medical devices. During that same a year, acupuncture was identified from the Countrywide Institutes of Health (NIH) for treating pain management and other medical ailments. The FDA presently regulates certain requirements for acupuncture needle usage and security.

## Obtaining Treated with Acupuncture

If you're considering treating your freak out symptoms through acupuncture, check with your physician; you need to obtain these services from a qualified acupuncturist. Professional acupuncture partitioners could be located through websites, just like the Countrywide Certification Commission rate for Acupuncture and Oriental Medication as well as the American Academy of Medical Acupuncture. Using acupuncture to deal with medical and mental medical issues continues to move up, rendering it more easily available; because it continues to be examined for effectiveness, which is obtainable through many hospitals; some plans may cover some of your acupuncture treatments.

Clinical trials examining acupuncture for anxiety show some positive results. However, this research has many restrictions, including small test sizes and limited methods to measure results. Acupuncturists and doctors are unclear about why it can benefit with anxiety and stress, but research has mentioned that acupuncture appears to have a relaxing impact. More rigorous scientific tests need to be carried out to have the ability to prove the potency of acupuncture for nervousness disorders.

Not all CAM practices have already been completely researched for protection and effectiveness; more information around the medical evidence, safeness, and risks of assorted CAM practices can be found in the Countrywide Middle for Complementary and Alternative Medication website. More standard treatment plans for panic disorders, such as for example medications and psychotherapy, have already been more supported by research. However, acupuncture could be considered a helpful addition to your standard treatment plan. Acupuncture could be the surplus treatment you'll need in reducing stress, and panic disorders symptoms.

## Health Advantages of Hearing Acupuncture

Hearing acupuncture is some sort of acupuncture which involves inserting needles into specific elements of the ear; revitalizing these factors is known to promote treating in the regions of the body referred to as auricular therapy or auricular-acupuncture, ear acupuncture is usually often incorporated into standard acupuncture treatments.

Although ear acupuncture is based on the principles of traditional Oriental medicine (some sort of alternative medicine that were only available in China), it started in the middle-20th century by French scientist Paul Nogier.

## Uses of Acupuncture

Acupuncture is reported to become useful in addressing several medical issues, including:

·    Anxiety.

·    Arthritis.

·    Persistent pain (such as for example headaches,

back pain, neck pain).

- Depression.

- Insomnia.

- Migraines.

- Nausea.

- Sciatica.

- Sinus congestion.

- Anxiety and stress.

- Tinnitus.

- Weight loss

Some individuals uses acupuncture to advertise fertility. Cosmetic acupuncture, also known as facial acupuncture, is useful to improve the appearance of skin.

Ear acupuncture is useful to improve the body's circulation of vital energy (also known as chi or qi) as well as to revive the equilibrium between yin and yang (two opposing but complementary energies) inside the inner organs. In traditional Chinese medicine, every one of these results is recognized as essential in working with disease and attaining health.

In alternative medicine, ear acupuncture is normally utilized for these and additional medical issues:

- Allergies.

- Anxiety.

- Arthritis.

- Chronic pain.

- Constipation.

- Depression.

- Fibromyalgia.

- Headaches.

- Insomnia.

- Irritable bowel syndrome.

- Low pain.

- Migraines

Furthermore, ear acupuncture could also be used to boost mood, help out with smoking cessation, alleviate pain, promote sounder rest, relieve stress, and support weight loss.

# Benefits

Although large-scale medical trials on ear acupuncture lack plenty of studies declare that this therapy may help out with treating several health issues. Listed below are many findings on ear acupuncture and its own potential health benefits.

## Insomnia

Many studies indicate that ear acupuncture might help relieve insomnia. These studies supported a released in Complementary Therapies in Medication in 2003, which tested the results of some sort of ear acupuncture, that involves using magnetic pearls to stimulate acupuncture points.

For the analysis, 15 seniors with insomnia were treated with hearing acupuncture for three weeks. Results exposed that folks experienced a considerable upsurge in both quality and degree of rest, with improvements enduring for half of a year after treatment ended.

## Smoking

Research on ear acupuncture's effectiveness like a smoking cessation support offers yielded combined results within a 2004 study released in the Swiss Journal of Research in Complementary and Natural Classical Medicine; for example, a survey of 126 individuals who had undergone ear acupuncture for smoking cessation found that the task had a one-year achievement rate of 41.1%. Predicated on the study's authors, this success rate makes hearing acupuncture "a competitive substitute for orthodox remedies withdrawal strategies."

In a written report published in the Journal from the American Board of Family Medicine, however, a trial involving 125 people found that ear acupuncture was far better than placebo treatment in enhancing the pace of smoking cessation. The analysis included five consecutive weeks of once-a-week treatments.

## Migraines

Ear canal acupuncture could be useful in treating migraines, according to a written report published in Acupuncture & Electro-Therapeutics Research in 2012. Analyzing findings on 35 migraine patients, the study's author determined that eight weeks of weekly ear acupuncture treatments led to significant improvements in pain and mood.

## Post-Surgery Pain

For any written report published in the Journal of Alternative and Complementary Medicine this season 2010, investigators sized up 17 studies on hearing acupuncture's performance in pain management. The report's authors figured ear acupuncture might flourish in treating various kinds of pain, especially postoperative pain.

## Constipation

Report review posted in the Journal of Alternative and Complementary Medicine this season 2010 demonstrates ear acupuncture may help out with treating constipation; for the review, researchers examined 29 studies on the use of ear acupuncture in constipation management.

Although all of the studies reported that ear acupuncture was effective in treating constipation, the writer review that because of significant flaws in the reviewed studies, even more research must confirm these findings.

**Using Hearing Acupuncture for Health**

If you're considering trying hearing acupuncture, make sure to consult a physician first. Self-treating and avoiding standard care can have serious consequences.

# Chapter 2

## How Does Acupuncture Work?

Acupuncture functions by stimulating the discharge of endorphins, your natural pain-relieving chemicals, in addition, it affects the autonomic nervous system as well as the release of chemicals that regulate blood flow and pressure, reduces swelling, and calm your brain.

## Advantages of Acupuncture

Some results from the available research on advantages of acupuncture are:

·      Low Back Pain

For any written report published in the annals of Internal Medicine in 2017, experts published the analyzed trials on the use of non-pharmacologic therapies (including acupuncture) for low back pain; the report authors found that acupuncture was connected with reduced pain strength and better function immediately after the acupuncture treatment, weighed against no acupuncture.

- Migraines

In 2016 review, released in the Cochrane Database of Systematic Reviews, researchers examined 22 previously released trials (involving 4985 individuals); of their summary, they found that adding acupuncture towards the treating of migraine symptoms may reduce the rate of recurrence; nevertheless, how big is the result is usually small in comparison to a sham acupuncture treatment.

- Tension Headaches

A 2016 review (involving 12 tests and 2349 individuals) demonstrates acupuncture involving at least six sessions might help people with standard tension of headaches. The analysts remember that the complete factors used during treatment may play a less important role than previously thought, which a lot of the power could be credited to needling results.

- Leg Pain

An analysis of previous post studies found that acupuncture improved physical function in individuals who have chronic knee pain, credited to osteoarthritis, nonetheless it appeared to provide just short-term (as much as 13 weeks) treatment.

Another review, posted in JAMA Surgery, analyzed non-pharmacological interventions for pain management after total knee arthroplasty and found evidence that acupuncture delayed the use of patient-controlled usage of opioid medication to ease pain.

AN AVERAGE Acupuncture Treatment is comparable to the original appointment; you will be asked to complete health history; the acupuncturist starts the visit by requesting about your overall health, diet, rest, stress level, along with other life-style practices. You may be asked about your feelings, appetite, food needs and wants, and reaction to adjustments in heat and cold seasons.

During your visit, the acupuncturist will test thoroughly your appearance carefully, being attentive to your tone, modulation of voice, and tongue color and covering. She or he will require your pulse at three factors on each wrist, noting the energy, quality, and tempo. In Chinese medication, the tongue and pulses are thought to reflect the fitness of the body organ systems and meridians.

Typically, acupuncture uses 6 to 15 tiny needles per treatment (the amount of needles doesn't indicate the intensity of the task). The needles ought to be left for 10 to 20 minutes; the acupuncturist may twist the needles for added impact.

Your acupuncturist might use additional techniques during your program, including:

Moxibustion: this may also be referred to as "moxa," moxibustion entails the use of warmed sticks (produced from dry out herbs) held near to the acupuncture needles to warm and stimulate the acupuncture factors.

Cupping: Glass mugs are placed on your own skin in order that there may be a suction impact. In TCM theory, cupping may be used to alleviate the stagnation of Qi and bloodstream.

Herbs: Chinese natural herbs could be gotten by from teas and pills.

Electro-acupuncture: A robust device is associated with

two to four acupuncture needles, providing a weak electric energy that stimulates the acupuncture needles through the procedure.

Laser acupuncture: that is utilized to activate acupuncture factors without the use of needles.

Ear acupuncture, also known as auricular acupuncture, could also be used through the procedure for weight-loss, smoking cessation, addictions, and anxiety.

Although the area from the acupuncture session varies from minutes to over 1 hour, the standard treatment length is 20 to 30 minutes; the initial visit usually takes around 60 minutes. Following a treatment, many people feel calm (as well as sleepy), although some experience energetic; in the event that you experience any uncommon symptoms, you need to talk to your doctor.

## Does Acupuncture Harm?

You may feel hook sting, pinch, ache, or some pain once the acupuncture needle is inserted; some acupuncturists change the acupuncture needle after it has been put into the torso, by twirling or revolving the needle, moving it along, or employing a machine with just a little electric pulse or current. Some acupuncturists consider the production of tingling, numbness, heavy feeling, or ache (referred to as "de Qi") preferred in achieving the therapeutic impact.

In the case whereby you have pain, numbness, or pain through the procedure, you must notify your acupuncturist immediately.

## UNWANTED EFFECTS of Acupuncture

Much like any treatment, acupuncture will pose some dangers like bleeding and pains immediately, plus the acupuncture needles are inserted. Additional undesirable effects range from epidermis rashes, allergies, bruising, pain, loss of blood, nausea, dizziness, fainting, or attacks.

To have the ability to slow up the risk of serious undesirable effects, acupuncture ought to be administered with a qualified and properly trained practitioner using sterile, disposable needles. According to some written report published in Scientific Reviews, acupuncture could cause unwanted severe effects, such as for example attacks, nerve and blood vessel injuries, problems from needle breakage or remnant needle items, punctured organs, central nervous system or spinal-cord injury,

hemorrhage, as well as other organ and cells injuries resulting in lack of life. Punctured pleural membranes round the lungs can lead to collapsed lungs. Individuals who have a distinctive, anatomical variance referred to as sternal foramen (an opening within the breastbone) are in risk of lung or center (pericardium) puncture.

There have been some reports of needles being left in following a treatment; a written statement released in the Bulletin of the World Health Business summarized the acupuncture-related undesirable effects in Oriental studies. Acupuncture is probably not right for folks with specific medical issues; the opportunity of loss of blood or bruising raises when you have a loss of blood disorder or are taking bloodstream thinners, such as for example warfarin (Coumadin).

# Chapter 3

## Acupuncture for Lowering High Blood Pressure

Around the 11th of June 2001, a lot of people swear by acupuncture; they said pincushion healed bad migraines or relentless again pain, others remain skeptical, dismissing the historical practice as mumbo jumbo. Now, researchers have started investigating the actions in coronary disease, and they found out not only that acupuncture works, but why and just how. They once informed WebMD that blood pressure medication may be replaced having a few pins and needles.

John C. Longhurst, MD, Ph.D., "I met an investigator who'd been undertaking work in acupuncture for a long period. I pointed out that he was an excellent scientist," he says. "I, similar to researchers, thought acupuncture was significant amounts of hocus pocus. However, once i noticed his work, I understood there is certainly something to it."

Long Hurst, a teacher of medication in the university of California, Irvine, University of Medicine, started four investigations in to the underlying systems of acupuncture; in it, his team tested cats with coronary disease. He said, "we demonstrated that acupuncture helped the pets by reducing ischemia, having less air to the guts" triggered when arteries are blocked; that was hard proof that the procedure worked well. Next, they attempted to regulate how it had been occurring.

Long Hurst says in acupuncture, the unseen pathways connecting one body part to another are called meridians. "They could be found over major [nerve] pathways that are accessed when you put a needle in." Rousing the pathway "sends impulses to your brain, activating different areas." Some influence pain, "which explains why acupuncture can control pain," he says, "aswell as others regulate the heart."

A definite area, just above the spinal-cord in your brain stem, regulates the discharge of adrenaline, a substance which makes the heart pound and blood pressure soar. However, if they induced, adrenaline in pets, and acupuncture avoided this from occurring. It blocked the effect," says Long Hurst. Hearts defeat usually, and blood pressure remained low.

In another examine, the team found they could invert acupuncture's heart-healthy effects by injecting cats using a synthetic version of naturally occurring opioids -- brain chemicals that induce a "runner's high," kicking in when we're in severe pain. "So, we're narrowing it down, getting more specific and comprehensive in conditions of what's happening," says Long Hurst.

Fourth research is underway in individual topics, he tells WebMD, but it's even now premature to attract any conclusions. The very best goal of the task is to greatly help the many patients with ischemia, high blood pressure, and irregular pulse, or heart arrhythmias, he tells WebMD. "The prevailing meds have a whole lot of side results; if we are able to reduce [their medication needed] with acupuncture, that will be great."

Experts agree it is not a far-fetched idea. "There have to be something even more to acupuncture compared to the placebo impact of hypnosis," says Joseph Alpert, MD,

Flinn Teacher of Medication and chairman from the division of medication at the faculty or university of Az in Tucson. "My co-workers have observed folks have exposed center surgery with only acupuncture, no anesthesia; this is not several malarkey," he tells WebMD, "it's real."

Pascal J. Goldschmidt, MD, FACC, principal of cardiology at Duke School, agrees that "It is not an accident that folks have been performing acupuncture for so very long," he tells WebMD. The email address details are "fairly obvious that it's not really a placebo impact. Acupuncture is apparently using a comparatively specific influence around the control of blood pressure."

## Acupuncture and Stroke

Strokes may appear to anyone from delivery through adulthood. You will find two different varieties of strokes; a stroke occurring when blood flow is about to forget travelling your brain is known as an ischemic heart stroke. A stroke occurring whenever a bloodstream vessel breaks or leaks at heart is named a hemorrhagic heart stroke. Both types of stroke are severe and, regarding the severity, could cause long-term damage; rehabilitation is definitely an essential part of coping with a heart stroke. As you could expect, rehabilitation options are enormous and cover from exercise to cognitive and psychological activities.

Some see acupuncture like a match to traditional treatment options. Continue reading to obtain additional on the huge benefits and dangers to getting acupuncture after a heart stroke.

## What exactly are the medical benefits of acupuncture?

Benefits

-       Acupuncture is usually a widely accepted alternative treatment for chronic pain.

-       It's also utilized to relax the body and mind.

Acupuncture is an Oriental healing practice that's around for a long time; it involves the use of slim, disinfected needles placed in to the epidermis by a professional acupuncturist. These needles sit in specific areas of the body that are believed to unleash various kinds of all-natural treating energy. For example, applying pressure towards the "third vision point" in the middle of your eyebrows is definitely thought to relieve headaches pain.

Although acupuncture is principally named an all-natural treatment for chronic pain, its potential benefits extend much beyond that; it has been used to aid in improving sleeping patterns and digestion of food. The practice, also, continues to be considered to relax the human brain and reduce stress or panic.

## What does the analysis say?

In one 2005 research, individuals who had experienced a stroke received the chance to try acupuncture therapy. The goal of the procedure was to greatly help reduce pain and discomfort due to the heart stroke. Experts discovered that people who received acupuncture noticed a noticable difference in wrist spasticity and flexibility in the wrist.

Although individuals who received acupuncture do see more development in comparison to those that didn't receive acupuncture, the quantity of improvement wasn't considered medically significant.

A lot more recent research demonstrates acupuncture in conjunction with exercise can succeed against make pain due to stroke.

More research is vital to determine whether acupuncture includes a definitive influence on recovery from stroke.

## What makes acupuncture work?

In the appointment, your acupuncturist will review your trouble and discuss just how they believe they'll assist you. Typically, they'll have a look at your tongue for more information about your overall health and consider your pulse.

When it's period for the task, they'll ask you to lay out; based on the region your acupuncturist will treat, you may be face up, face down, or working out for you. Your acupuncturist will softly devote sterile, single-use needles in the areas they believe your body will take benefit of the most.

You will likely feel them inserting the needles; nevertheless, you almost certainly won't experience any pain. During this time period, your acupuncturist may bring high temperatures or massage therapy to your therapy.

One program typically lasts 30 mins. An average span of acupuncture therapy requires up to 12 classes. Some insurance firms cover the trouble of acupuncture therapy, so be sure to check with your supplier about your alternatives.

## Dangers and Warnings

Risks

-      The using unsterilized needles could cause health complications.

-      You might encounter bruising or bleeding over the injection sites.

Before seeing an acupuncturist, visit a medical doctor and discuss your desire to add acupuncture to your recovery plan. They are able to assist you to evaluate whether this is actually the most suitable decision for you personally. Acupuncture is probably not for you when you have a loss of blood disorder or if you're taking bloodstream thinners.

After consulting a medical doctor, research acupuncturists locally; make sure that they're certified and pursuing all health rules.

After your appointment, you may experience loss of blood, bruising, or soreness on the insertion sites. That is clearly a standard response to the task. If you begin experiencing any uncommon symptoms, you should talk to your doctor.

## Alternatives to Acupuncture

If you're no applicant for acupuncture or want to try traditional means of treatment, you have many other choices. Based on your requirements, you may receive inpatient or outpatient treatment. This may consist of conversation, occupational, and physical therapy. These treatments might help you to regain the use of your talk, aswell as the amount of movements in the hands, lower limbs, and hands.

If the mind was damaged during your stroke, you may even have to go to a neurologist for a lot more treatment. It might also be good to consult a psychiatrist. They are able to help you straighten out your feelings as you navigate your recovery.

# Chapter 4

## The Acupuncture Factors for Legs

*Chinese medicine theory believes your energy, or Qi, circulates through energy channels called meridians. These meridians match the inner organs, which are believed to govern their vigour stream; many meridians run the length from the legs, the belly, spleen, gallbladder, kidney, and liver organ channels; stimulating several factors to produce a difference in decreasing the leg health. Pain, weakness, and numbness could be suffering from needling or pressing specific calf points.*

## Acupuncture

## What to learn about an Acupuncture Appointment;

*Get hold of your doctor prior to trying acupuncture, particularly if you possess medical ailments that impact your circulatory and nervous systems. A qualified acupuncturist begins by requesting about your wellbeing background, collecting current and past info to make a Chinese medication diagnosis; she'll also ask to look at your tongue, consider your pulse on both wrists and discuss her meant treatment plan; thin needles will be placed into assorted places, and leave place for between 10 and 45 minutes. During this time period, you are able to relax and meditate while hearing music, and even rest. In the event that you might feel instantaneous results, several or higher sessions are often recommended to control your conditions properly.*

## Meridians around the Legs

*Vigour meridians run along the trunk and edges of the legs, surrounding your leg and ankle bones, as well as addressing your toes; it could be indicated for local treatment dysfunctions within the spot surrounding the theory. Besides, they serve additional functions, such as for example alleviating pain, numbness and bloating, increasing energy, or balancing feelings. The spleen route can impact muscle power, quality of bloodstream, and bloat. Belly meridian factors can move energy blocks and decrease pain, while kidney factors can increase energy and reduce warmth; the liver organ and gallbladder stations inspire feelings like anger, bloodstream disorders, and menstrual problems.*

## Factors In charge of Pain or Swelling

*For pain and swelling from the legs, your practitioner may choose kidney point 1, spleen 6, gallbladder 40 and 41 or liver organ 3. Kidney 1 can be found on each and every foot, helping restore essential energy and strength while reducing pain and bloating. Gallbladder 40 and 41 spread power, focusing on pain in the hips and calves. Spleen 6 might help regulate dampness, resolving bloating round the inner rearfoot area.*

## Numbness and Weakness

*Numbness and weakness in the lower limbs could be regulated by stimulating gallbladder factors 29 and 31, as well as abdomen 33 and 37, kidney 1 and 9, and bladder 40 or 58. Located in the hip will be the external thigh and leading thigh areas, respectively, gallbladder 29, 31, and tummy 33 are indicated for numbness or weakness in the reduced extremities. Kidney 9 and belly 37 can be found within the weak knee, while bladder 40 and 58 can be found near the again from the leg and leg, respectively. Every one of these factors can decrease pain, numbness, and weakness in the lower limbs.*

## Acupuncture & Hormone Balance

*Although acupuncture may not seem as being a reasonable choice for hormonal imbalances, it might incorporate some benefits. Acupuncture is usually part of traditional Oriental medication TCM, which includes inserting slim needles into specific factors of your body. The elements match different organs whose energy operates along with stations called meridians. Regarding TCM theory, stimulating factors might help restore healthy balance to your body. Get hold of your doctor about acupuncture; look for a professional Oriental practitioner to debate your hormonal balance.*

## Inserting Acupuncture Needles

## Hormones

*Hormones play essential functions in a vast collection of functions within you, including metabolism, duplication, and sleep-wake cycles. Associated with traditional western medical technology, hormones are secreted by glands in the mind and body, just like the pituitary and adrenal glands; they travel via the bloodstream to various cells to execute their jobs. Although much emphasis is put on sex hormones like estrogen and testosterone, thyroid and adrenal hormones are simply like essential to ideal health.*

## Chinese Theory

*Acupuncture.com says that Chinese medication considers hormones to be a part of someone's Jing, or substance. You receive birth to an amount of life pressure, or fact, which is kept in your kidney, and used throughout your lifetime to nourish cells and organs. Jing includes blood and liquids, and yang, such as energy and warmness. Predicated on the web site, when substance depletes, its experience is comparable to hormonal imbalances, such as for example menopause or impotence; Oriental medicine treatments focus on factors that may restore fact; organs just like the kidneys as well as the liver organ will also be associated with hormone balance.*

# Kidney

*In "A Manual of Acupuncture" by Peter Deadman, the kidney is known as being the building blocks of life within you. It stores your substance and dominates duplication and development. Because Traditional western medication believes hormones to test an enormous role in these methods, your Chinese specialist range from kidney acupuncture factors within your hormone-balancing treatment. In March 2010, the "Journal of Traditional Oriental Medicine" featured a written report that investigated the results of specific acupuncture stage activation for the reproductive hormone gonadotropin-releasing hormone. The analysis found that the kidney's vigour collection, or meridian, performed employment in revitalizing the discharge from the hormone; kidney level 10 experienced a substantial influence on release.*

## Liver/Gallbladder

*The liver organ and gallbladder is a set of yin-yang, according to Chinese medicine theory as the yin body organ, the liver organ stores and keeps bloodstream and governs a woman's menstrual period; the gallbladder excretes yang action bile for the break down of food. The analysis in the "Journal of Traditional Chinese Medication" also lists gallbladder and liver organ points as positively revitalizing the discharge of gonadotropin-releasing hormone. Gallbladder factors 26 and 34, as well as liver organ factors 14, were outlined.*

## Ren/Du Channels

*The ren route can be referred to as the conception vessel, associated with Deadman's publication, whose factors work to harmonize disorders within their geographic area. The route works along the midline of leading of the body, which is often used to deal with infertility of men and women, and help out with menopausal issues. The du route, referred to as the regulating vessel, moves along the midline from the trunk of the body; "A Manual of Acupuncture" claims it mediates in the middle of your brain and the guts. In circumstances of reproductive hormone excitement, conception vessel factors four and 17 were detailed in the analysis in "Journal of Traditional*

*Chinese Medication," along with regulating vessel three.*

# Chapter 5

## 6 Pressure Factors for Anxiety Relief

*Understanding anxiety*

Lots of people experience stress within their everyday living; you might experience moderate symptoms when facing a challenging or nerve-racking position. You might have more severe, long-lasting symptoms that impact your way of life, including:

·       Feelings of stress, dread, or worry.

·       Restlessness.

·       Difficulty concentrating.

·       Difficulty drifting off to sleep or staying asleep.

·       Fatigue.

·       Irritability.

·       Nausea, headaches, or digestive concerns.

- Feeling inadequate control.

- Muscle tension.

Anxiety is normally treated with therapy, medication, or an assortment of both. There's also many treatments, including acupressure, which can only help.

Acupressure is some sort of traditional Chinese medication that may provide temporary rest from panic symptoms; it needs revitalizing pressure factors within you, either on your own or with a professional.

Six pressure factors you can attempt for anxiety alleviation.

1. Hall of impression point

The hall of impression point is based on the center of your eyebrows; applying pressure until now is considered to help with both anxiety and stress.

To utilize this aspect:

- Sit comfortably; it will help you to close your eye also.

· Touch the positioning between your eyebrows together with your index finger or thumb.

· Consider decrease, deep breaths, and apply gentle, company pressure inside a round movement for 5 to 10 minutes.

2. Heavenly gate point

The heavenly gate point can be found in the very best shell of the ear, by the end from the triangle-like hollow there. Stimulating this aspect is thought to support relieve anxiousness, stress, and insomnia.

To utilize this aspect:

· Locate the theory within your ear; it might help make use of a reflection.

· Apply company, gentle pressure within a round motion for two minutes.

3. Make good point

The shoulder well point is at your shoulder muscle. To believe it pinches your muscle together with your middle finger and thumb. This pressure point is thought to assist with reducing stress, muscle tension, and headaches. Additionally, it could stimulate labor, so don't use this stage if you're pregnant.

To utilize this aspect:

· Find the theory on your help to make muscle.

· Pinch the muscle together with your thumb and middle finger.

· Apply gentle, firm pressure together with your index finger and massage the theory for four to five seconds.

· Release the pinch as you massage therapy the point.

4. Union valley point

You get this pressure level between your thumb and index finger. Stimulating this aspect is considered to reduce stress, headaches, and neck pain. Similar to the shoulder wellpoint, additionally, it could induce labor, so avoid this aspect if you're pregnant.

To utilize this aspect:

·　　Together with your index finger and thumb, apply firm pressure towards the webbing in the middle of your thumb and index finger of the other hand.

·　　Massage the pressure point for four to five seconds, taking decrease, deep breaths.

5. Great surge point

The great surge pressure point is on your own foot, about several finger widths below the intersection of the big toe and second toe; the theory is dependant on the hollow just above the bone.

This pressure point can help lessen anxiety and stress; you can also put it to use for pain, insomnia, and menstrual cramps.

To utilize this aspect:

·　　Find the theory by moving your finger down along from between your 1st two toes.

·　　Apply company, deep pressure to the theory.

- Therapeutic massage for four to five a few moments.

6. Internal frontier gate point

You will discover the inner frontier gate point on your own arm, around three finger widths below your wrist. Revitalizing this aspect can help to lessen anxiety and stress, also reducing nausea and pain.

To utilize this aspect:

- Turn one hand which means that your palm faces up.

- Togethe with your additional hand, measure three hands below your wrist. The theory can be found here, in the hollow in the middle of your tendons.

Apply pressure to the theory and massage therapy for four to five seconds.

The analysis behind acupressure for anxiety

There's limited research about the use of acupressure and pressure factors for concern. But experts are starting to take a look at alternative anxiety treatments.

Most of the studies that do exist have devoted to pressure factors for nervousness before a potentially stressful situation or medical procedure, instead of general stress.

For example, a 2015 summary of many studies examining the results of acupressure on anxiety found that acupressure seemed to help relieve stress before a medical procedure such as for example surgery.

Another 2015 research of 85 people hospitalized for malignancy treatment found that acupressure helped to reduce their anxiety.

A 2016 study viewed anxiety in 77 students with severe menstrual pain. Acupressure applied at the great surge pressure point during three menstrual cycles reduced stress in research participants by the final of another cycle.

A 2018 research found that acupressure helped reduce anxiety and stress symptoms in women getting fertility treatments.

Much bigger studies saw a company grip on how best to employ pressure factors for anxiety. However, the prevailing studies haven't found any unwanted side effects of acupressure on panic symptoms, so that it may be worth a chance if you're wanting to consider using new approaches.

Just retain at heart these studies also declare that acupressure seems to provide temporary rest from symptoms. Make sure to match all of the stress management, therapy, or other treatments recommended by a medical doctor while attempting acupressure.

## Know when to see a doctor

While acupressure may provide some short-term rest from anxiety symptoms, there's hardly any proof that it'll help with long-term anxiety.

If you realise that your anxiety symptoms are developing, rendering it hard to go to work or college or even to hinder your associations, maybe it's time to talk with physician or therapist - concerned about the price tag on therapy? Listed here are therapy choices for every budget.

You should talk with physician or therapist in the event

that you begin to see:

- Emotions of depression.

- Thoughts of suicide.

- Panic attacks.

- Trouble sleeping.

- Headaches.

- digestive problems

## Acupuncture for PANIC DISORDERS

Complementary and substitute medicine (CAM) is regarded as many unconventional practices and products used to advertise health insurance and therapeutic. Lately, CAM strategies have grown to be popular; to take care of mental medical issues, including depressive disorder, post-traumatic stress disorder (PTSD), and various other anxiousness disorders. Some typically standard CAM procedures include intensifying muscle rest, aromatherapy, pilates, and therapeutic massage.

Acupuncture is a different kind of CAM practice that may enhance personal wellbeing. Considered among the very most popular types of CAM, acupuncture is actually being used to deal with a range of circumstances. As acupuncture keeps growing in recognition, more research has been devoted to this treatment for the panic symptoms.

## The 5 Best Acupuncture Factors for Anxiety

Nothing diminishes panic faster than an action quote; there are always a large numbers of acupuncture factors for anxiety. Stress could be treated with a massive collection of acupuncture period combinations based on the main pattern, which is exclusive to every individual. However, these five acupuncture factors for anxiousness represent the ones I benefit from most in my own clinic; predicated on your specific symptoms and encounters like a person, your treatment changes. These factors can help your anxiety and stress and will most likely change from treatment to treatment as your symptoms change.

Acupuncture factors help treat nervousness by activating the nervous system, specifically the parasympathetic nervous system, which reduces cortisol stress hormones. Acupuncture also produces endorphins, natural pain-killing opioids, and other feel-good chemicals at heart. Chronic stress creates deep neural pathways which may be hard to boost. By spending 1-2 hours weekly in conditions of rest, you are assisting in creating a fresh neural pathway and stopping reinforcing the panic tract. Medications for anxiousness have a tendency to exist highly addictive and possess dangerous drawbacks symptoms, such as for example severe rebound anxiety and stress.

Acupuncture is capable of doing long-lasting results without adverse part effects.

1. Heart 7

This point can be found within the ulnar side from the wrist and works to calm the Shen, or "spirit." If we possess repressed feelings or sleepless evenings, and even if we desire vividly we may include an imbalance called "Heart Open fire" in Traditional Oriental Medication; other symptoms of centerfire including, race center, palpitations or center flutters, sweating at night time, high blood pressure, red-tipped tongue, and red face. This imbalance is treated by calming the guts, which Centre 7 does superbly.

## 2. Regulating Vessel 24du 20 and du 24 acupuncture factors for anxiety

This point can be found just inside the hairline in the heart from the forehead. It works to relax the anxious system by sending energy down.

Race thoughts and "monkey brain" make it hard to relax, which acupuncture points helps immediately that anxious energy down and out.

## 3. Pericardium 6

This point can be found inside the wrist, about 3 inches from your crease. It really is accessible for assisting with nausea and a lot of the magnetic bracelets sold for car and sea sickness work by stimulating this aspect. Furthermore, to cope with nausea, this aspect opens the chest muscles and the guts. The pericardium may be the protector of the guts, and sometimes if we are stressed, we are overprotected and guarded. This aspect counteracts the contracting energy of nervousness.

Shenmen acupuncture factors for anxiety4.

## 4. Shenmen

This aspect is put in the ear; ear factors might appear scary; however, they have become relaxing; this aspect calms the soul by helping the body become parasympathetic or "rest and breakdown" mode. Instead of "battle or air travel" setting, activating the parasympathetic system causes cortisol stress hormones to drop, reducing anxiety. Ear factors easily access the central anxious system as the nerves go directly to the brain center.

Yintang acupuncture factors for anxiety

## 5. Yintang

The best from the acupuncture points for anxiety is situated in the middle of your brows. In Hinduism and yoga exercises, that is known as the 3rd vision; this area can be found for the pineal gland, which helps control melatonin. Melatonin is a hormone in charge of restful rest and healthy rest/wake cycles; this aspect is uniquely powerful at coping with insomnia, due to overthinking.

# Chapter 6

## Acupuncture for Digestive Problems

Released July 18, 2017, by Hailin Wu, OM Clinical / Faculty Supervisor, Program Director & filed under Acupuncture and Massage College.

Acupuncture for digestive problems is an efficient and safe way to naturally treat many acute and chronic conditions from the vital body. If you have attempted conventional medication to keep digestive issues in balance without success, consider acupuncture, which can be an alternative health treatment without part effects.

Acupuncture can help in treating many digestive disorders, including:

· Bacterial infections.

· Peptic ulcers.

· Heartburn.

- Lactose intolerance.

- Gastrointestinal tract bleeding.

- Inflammatory conditions.

- Hiatus hernia syndrome

## What makes acupuncture treatment help?

Using acupuncture for digestive problems functions by nourishing related organs, reducing irritation from the belly and pancreas, and enhancing digestive functions. Throughout treatment, the specialist will identify certain acupuncture factors on your own body, usually the ones that speed up metabolism, increase gastrointestinal muscle contraction and rest, reduce gastric acid secretion, and control small and large intestine function, and restores abdomen acidity on the right track levels.

Together with Oriental herbal medicine and stress reduction techniques, acupuncture for digestive problems pays in treating general gastrointestinal symptoms.

Furthermore, to acupuncture for digestive problems, moxibustion - a way of applying the herb mugwort to acupuncture factors - may also be utilized as an anti-inflammatory agent and to notify imbalances. Individuals often experience long-term symptomatic comfort with acupuncture for digestive problems, aswell as reduced stress and improved energy.

Acupuncture for digestive problems may integrate ideas for life-style modifications to have the ability to correct diet imbalances and regulate digestion of food. The World Health Corporation identifies acupuncture for digestive issues as an efficient treatment for digestive imbalance.

## The Resources of Digestive Disorders

Digestion disorders could be the result of a number of factors, such as for example chronic stress and other nutritional issues, such as for example overeating or eating so many high-fat foods. Acupuncture can treat digestive imbalance by reducing stress and regulating the endocrine and anxious system hyperactivity that often accompanies digestive disorder patterns.

Acupuncture is a remedy that may be built-into allopathic or holistic healthcare seamlessly. Acupuncture for digestive problems can be an all-natural health maintenance therapy.

## Acupuncture and Abdomen Disorders

We are often asked this question every time a conversation arises about tummy disorders and acupuncture; ''can acupuncture support me personally in order to avoid needing antacids regularly?'' or "think about my acid reflux disorder?"

Individuals are amazed once We clarify to them that acupuncture can treat most gastrointestinal issues such as for example acid reflux disorder, bloating, and indigestion very effectively.

According to Oriental Medicine, the Belly is usually a significant standard (organ) within our body. It really is so essential that there's a custom of acupuncture that concentrates mainly around the Stomach (and its particular 'sister body organ' the Spleen). If the Belly cannot function to its fullest capacity in comparison with someone who struggles to become wholly nourished within their Body, Brain, or Spirit.

The Stomach is vital so you can get our food nourishment (or GuQi) and in addition our mental and spirit level nourishment. We must process info (i.e., might know about read, study, pay attention to, discover, etc.) which work includes our belly. We also have to receive and procedure psychological materials, which also involves our abdomen.

A whole lot of my patients who are in university or graduate frequently have Stomach issues, that have mostly resolved with acupuncture and vanished once they complete their studies. I've treated many individuals who have medical diagnoses of acid reflux disorder; these circumstances, along with problems like belching, hiccupping, as well as nausea, are categorized as the band of Rebellious Stomach Qi. When the Stomach becomes weakened or stressed or out of balance the Qi may rise, that leads towards the symptoms mentioned previously (rebellious Stomach). You will see multiple points and treatment possibilities to deal with stomach disorders. Remember, the Stomach is among the most extended meridians on your own body; they have 45 points about it. Combine that using the interplay of other 'Officials' on your own body (as I'll elaborate below), and an acupuncturist should come up with multiple treatment plans for you personally.

Many fundamental imbalances in the body can lead to 'rebellious stomach Qi.' For example, the Liver Standard (or meridian) is in charge of the clean flow of feelings (according to Chinese medicine). If we are chronically stressed or tense/anxious/angry/ depressed, etc., our Liver Standard may begin to impact onto the Stomach resulting in the Stomach to 'rebel.' How many times you might have noticed someone cry 'I can't stomach it anymore' they could lose their appetite. A lot of people may gain in appetite.

Another cause could possibly be linked to the Kidney Recognized (or meridian). Regarding Chinese Medication, among the products the Kidney does is help warm the organs so they can function optimally. Sometimes, with age, the Kidney Official weakens and has less capacity to warm the body; this might cause the Stomach to decline response. I'm sure you have found out about the elderly complaining of more difficulty in digesting different varieties of food auspices because they age. Or, they are able to forget about eat large meals-when smaller, more frequent meals are better tolerated.

Many people complain of an even more generalized symptom of 'sensitive stomach.' They present with bloating and gas, making their waistbands feel tight after meals. Often these people report an exceptionally long history of the symptoms. The sign may occasionally arrive if they are really stressed about something within their life. Or it becomes their 'check engine light' reminding them that they need to practice some of the fresh coping strategies they've learned within their acupuncture journey. The symptom has resolved to the level where it is the exception instead of the rule within their life. Simply, acupuncture offers helped them to gain access to the central point where they are able to manage their stomach instead of it controlling them.

Do you realize the belly functions at its best if we ingest warm food; iced drinks, cold foods, freezing desserts, actually stress the stomach, food that's too spicy may also put strain on the stomach after a while. Our diet program over our lifetime can eventually contribute to the weakening of our stomach after we age. An acupuncturist is trained to greatly help identify what's stressing your stomach in order that lifestyle changes could be suggested.

Aswell as the annals you provide to your acupuncturist, the pulse reading as well as the tongue evaluation offer valuable information in identifying the fitness of your stomach. This assists in formulating a remedy plan that's created for you.

Keep the Belly in mind when you ingest meals. It doesn't like being overly stuffed, which burdens the Abdomen. So, eat slower, laugh a whole lot, consider smaller portions, don't drink cold beverages together with your meal (sip on room temperature water instead), and consume throughout the day.

# Chapter 7

## How to use Pressure Factors to alleviate Headaches

- There are many popular pressure points in the body considered to relieve headaches. Here's where they might be and methods to use them:

- Union valley

- The union valley points are available on the web between your thumb and index finger. To deal with headaches:

- - Start by pinching this region using the thumb and index finger of the reverse hands firmly - however, not painfully - for 10 seconds.

- - Next, make small circles together with your thumb upon this field in one direction for ten a few moments each.

- - Continue doing this technique around the

Union Valley stage on your own contrary hand.

- This type of pressure point treatment is considered to relieve tension in the very best and neck. The pressure is often connected with headaches.

- Drilling bamboo

- Drilling bamboo factors are available in the indentations on either facet of the spot that the bridge of the nose area matches the ridge of the eyebrows. To employ these pressure factors to take care of headaches:

- · Usage both of the index hands to use company pressure to both elements simultaneously.

- · Hold for 10 seconds.

- · Release and repeat.

- Pressing these pressure factors can relieve headaches that are triggered by eye strain and sinus pain or pressure.

- Gates of consciousness

- The gates of consciousness pressure points are available in the bottom from the skull in the parallel hollow areas in the middle of your two vertical neck muscles. To apply these pressure factors:

- · Place your index and middle hands of either hand onto these pressure factors.

- · Press firmly upward on both edges simultaneously for ten a few moments, then release and repeat

- · Applying strong touch to these pressure factors might help reduce headaches triggered by tension in the neck.

- Third eye

- THE 3RD eye point comes in the center of your two eyebrows, where in fact the bridge of the nose meets your forehead.

- Make use of the index finger of just one 1 hand to

use firm pressure to the region for 1 minute.

- Firm pressure placed on the 3rd attention pressure stage is considered to alleviate eyestrain and sinus pressure that often causes headaches.

- Shoulder well

- The shoulder well can be found at the edge of your shoulder, halfway between your shoulder point and underneath of the neck. To make use of this usually pressure point:

- · Utilize the thumb of just 1 hand to use firm, round pressure until now for 1 minute.

- · Then change and repeat on the other hand side.

- Applying solid touch towards the produce good pressure point might help alleviate stiffness within your neck

# Chapter 8

## Cluster Headaches

Cluster headaches are some relatively brief but excruciating headaches each day for weekly or weeks at exactly the same time; you have a tendency to get them at the same time each year, just like the springtime or fall. For his or her seasonal character, people often mistake cluster headaches for symptoms of allergies or business stress.

We've no idea the causes of them, but we are able to say for certain a nerve for the reason that person is involved, creating extreme pain around among your eyes. It's so awful that the majority of people can't sit back nonetheless and may often speed during an assault. Cluster headaches may become more severe in comparison with a migraine; however, they often don't last for long.

They are minimal common types of headaches, affecting less than 1 in 1,000 people. Men keep these things a lot more than women do; you usually begin to have them before generation 30. Cluster headaches may vanish completely (enter remission) for any couple of months or years; however, they are able to keep coming back again without the caution.

## What Happens

You get yourself a cluster headache every time a specific nerve pathway in the mind is activated; that transmission appears to derive from a deeper section of the brain called the hypothalamus, where, actually, the "internal natural clock" that handles your rest and wake cycles lives.

The nerve that's affected is recognized as the trigeminal nerve, and it's in charge of sensations such as for example temperature or pain for the reason that person. It's near your eyesight, and its own branches up to your forehead, across your cheek, down your jaw range, and above your hearing about the same side, too. A root brain condition, just like a tumor or aneurysm, won't cause these headaches.

## Characteristics of Cluster Headaches

Many things get this to sort of headache different. They include:

· Speed: Cluster headaches generally reach their full push quickly; within 5 or ten minutes.

· Pain: It's generally, one-sided, and it remains about the same side within a period, plenty of time if you're getting daily shows. Whenever a fresh headache period begins, it might switch to the contrary part, but that's uncommon; it could be throbbing or constant. You'll look it behind or using one eye; it might spread to your forehead, temple, nasal, cheek, or top gum on that aspect, your mind could be sensitive, you could feel your bloodstream pulsing.

· Brief duration: Cluster headaches usually only last 30 to 90 minutes; they may be as short as quarter-hour or so long as 3 hours, however they disappear. You may most probably obtain someone who experience among three from the headaches every day, however, many individuals have just one another day, although some keep these things up to 8 occasions per day.

· Predictable: Attacks look like from your circadian tempo, your 24-hour clock. They happen so regularly, generally at exactly the same time every day, they may be called "noisy alarms headaches." They might even wake you up a few hours after you fall asleep. Night time episodes may become more serious than daytime ones.

· Frequent: Lots of people will definitely get day-by-day headaches for two weeks to 90 days; among these periods, they'll be pain-free for at least 2 weeks.

Symptoms

The pain usually starts suddenly. When occurring, you might see:

· Pain or a mild burning sensation.

· Swollen or drooping eye.

· Smaller pupil in the interest.

· Eye inflammation or watering.

· Runny or congested nose.

· Red and warm face.

· Sweating.

·     You're private to light

Cluster headaches are more frequent in individuals who smoke or are heavy drinkers. Within a cluster period, you'll be even more delicate to alcohol consumption and nicotine; simply little alcohol consumption can lead to headaches.

## Possible Causes and Triggers

When you're in the heart of a cluster period, these may bring around the headache:

·     Cigarette smoke.

·     Alcohol.

·     Strong smells

Treatment

You have several choices when it comes to treating these headaches

Medications

- Acute stroke treatments: This can help when the headaches hit.

- Triptans: These drugs are among the improved ways to look after the pain. You'll find:

Sumatriptan (Alsuma, Imitrex, Sumavel), which works both as a chance or inhaled

Zolmitriptan (Zomig)

Dihydroergotamine (D.H.E. 45): This prescription drug would depend within the ergot fungus.

- Lidocaine: That is a pain reliever, employing a nose spray.

- Oxygen: A medical doctor might call it inhaled oxygen. You'll breathe it in through a nose and mouth mask for quarter-hour.

Preventive medicine could stop a headache before it starts, a medical doctor can prescribe medication to shorten the area from the cluster as well as lessen the severity of the attacks, including:

- Corticosteroid, like prednisone, for some time.

- Sodium (Depakene, Depakote).

- Ergotamine tartrate (Cafergot, Ergomar).

- Gabapentin.

- Carbonate

- Topiramate (Qudexy XR, Topamax, Trokendi XR)

- Verapamil (Calan, Covera, Verelan)

Occipital nerve end (a medical doctor may possibly also call it occipital nerve injection): The physician will inject a number of anesthetic and steroids into these nerves. Located in the bottom of the skull, they're usually the place to start for headaches; that is clearly a short-term treatment until a precautionary will start to work.

Nerve Activation: A lot of people who don't respond to medication have better fortune with:

Occipital nerve stimulation: A medical doctor surgically implants an instrument that sends electric impulses towards the band of nerves in the bottom of the skull.

Neuromodulator: These FDA-approved noninvasive devices include:

Cefaly: You put electrodes on your own forehead and connect these to a headband-like controller that sends indicators to your supraorbital nerve.

Gamma-Core: This product, also known as a noninvasive vague nerve stimulator (NVNS), uses electrodes to send indicators towards the nerve.

Surgery

If nothing else works, surgery could be a choice for those who don't get an escape from cluster headaches. Deep brain stimulation which involves putting an electrode deep in the mind is losing choose to less invasive options.

Most methods involve blocking the trigeminal nerve, an initial pathway for pain. It sets the spot around your eyes, but a misstep can cost weakness within your jaw and insufficient feeling for the reason that person and head.

# Lifestyle Changes

These moves can help you avoid cluster headaches:

Keep a normal sleep plan: A substantial change to your program can begin a headache.

Skip alcohol consumption: Any type, even ale, and wines can trigger a bout of headaches when you're inside a cluster series.

# Alternative Treatments

Capsaicin: A nose spray from the pain reliever can help.

Melatonin: This medication, known for easing sleep issues like aircraft lag, might lower the amount of headaches.

# Acknowledgements

The Glory of this book success goes to God Almighty and my beautiful Family, Fans, Readers & well-wishers, Customers, and Friends for their endless support and encouragement.